Perfect Italian Pasta"75 Recipes for Beginner-Proof Italian First Courses"

Foreword by Giorgio Sapori

Dear readers,Pasta is the soul of Italian cuisine, a dish that for centuries has brought families together, celebrated special occasions, and brought joy even to the most ordinary days. This book stems from my passion for the culinary tradition of our country and the desire to share with you 75 recipes that tell the story of Italy, region by region, flavor by flavor.Each recipe is designed to be simple, accessible, and foolproof because I believe that cooking should not be complicated but a rewarding experience for everyone, beginners and experts alike. Whether you're passionate about classic sauces like Amatriciana, devotees of the perfect Carbonara, lovers of homemade fresh pasta, or explorers of modern and creative flavors, here you'll find something that will win you over.While writing this book, I wanted to include not only the techniques and ingredients but also the little secrets that make all the difference in cooking: freshly hand-torn basil, the choice of a good extra virgin olive oil, or the art of cooking pasta always al dente.Italian cuisine is an invaluable heritage, and pasta is its beating heart. With this book, I hope to take you on a journey of authentic flavors, genuine ingredients, and a deep love for the table. Grab a pot, a pinch of curiosity, and let your palate guide you.Happy cooking and, above all, buon appetito! With affection,Giorgio Sapori

"Welcome to the magical world of Italian pasta!"If there's one dish that represents Italy around the world, it's pasta. Simple in its ingredients but extraordinarily versatile, pasta is the beating heart of thousands of recipes that tell stories of tradition, innovation, and passion. This recipe book is designed for anyone who wants to approach the world of Italian cuisine, even starting from scratch.Our goal is to make every recipe accessible and foolproof. We've created detailed instructions, explaining every step—from selecting ingredients to cooking times—so that even those who have never cooked can achieve restaurant-worthy results.In addition to learning how to prepare traditional classic dishes, you'll discover how to reinvent flavors with a personal touch. Each recipe is enriched with practical tips, suggestions for variations, and little tricks that make all the difference.Get ready to transform your kitchen into a little corner of Italy. With "Perfect Pasta," every dish will be a journey through authentic flavors and love for good food.Ready to start? Put on your apron and set the water to boil: perfect pasta awaits you!

Introduction to Italian Pasta Pasta is much more than just food: it's a symbol of conviviality, tradition, and culture. It is loved in every corner of the world, but its roots lie at the heart of Italy, where every region boasts its own recipes and variations. In this chapter, we will explore the history of pasta, its basic ingredients, and its main types, giving you a solid foundation to successfully tackle all the recipes in this book.

The History of Pasta The origins of pasta are shrouded in mystery and legend. Although many associate the introduction of pasta in Italy with Marco Polo's journey to China, this theory has been debunked by numerous historians. It is instead believed that the ancient Romans already knew a primitive form of pasta called "lagana."The production of dried pasta, as we know it today, developed in Southern Italy thanks to the ideal climate for drying the dough made from durum wheat and water. From Naples to Sicily, pasta became a staple food for Italian families before spreading throughout the rest of the country and the world.

The Fundamental Ingredients Pasta is distinguished by its simplicity: only two basic ingredients are needed for its production. However, the quality of these ingredients is essential to achieving an excellent result.

- **Flour or durum wheat semolina:**Traditional Italian pasta is made with durum wheat semolina, which gives a firm texture and a unique ability to hold sauces. Soft wheat flour, on the other hand, is mainly used for fresh pasta.

- **Water:**Only water and semolina are needed to create most dried pasta. In fresh pasta, eggs are often added to obtain an elastic and rich dough.In some regional recipes, like potato gnocchi, alternative ingredients come into play, but simplicity and purity remain constant.

Types of Pasta In Italy, there are hundreds of pasta shapes, each with its ideal use. Here's an overview of the main types:

- **Long pasta:** spaghetti, linguine, tagliatelle, fettuccine.Perfect with creamy or simple sauces, like pesto or carbonara.

- **Short pasta:** penne, rigatoni, fusilli, farfalle.Ideal for holding thick and hearty sauces like ragù.
- **Stuffed pasta:** ravioli, tortellini, agnolotti.Little pockets of goodness, often filled with meat, vegetables, or cheeses.
- **Baked pasta:** lasagna, cannelloni.Perfect for rich, layered dishes, ideal for special occasions.

Choosing the Pasta When buying pasta, look for products made with high-quality durum wheat semolina. To recognize it, observe the surface: high-quality pasta has a rough appearance, perfect for absorbing sauces. Also, always read the cooking instructions: the recommended time is a good indicator of the texture you'll achieve.As for fresh pasta, if you're not making it at home, choose artisanal varieties, which have a more authentic texture than industrial ones.

Storing Pasta

- **Dried pasta:** Store it in a cool, dry place, away from direct light and humidity. If stored properly, it can last for years.

- **Fresh pasta:** It should be kept in the refrigerator and consumed within a few days. You can also freeze it, but make sure to protect it well to prevent it from drying out.

A Journey Through Italian Regions Each Italian region has its own typical pasta and emblematic recipes. Here are a few examples:

- **Lazio:** spaghetti alla carbonara, bucatini all'amatriciana.
- **Liguria:** trofie al pesto.
- **Campania:** paccheri with Neapolitan ragù.
- **Emilia-Romagna:** lasagna alla bolognese, tortellini in broth.
- **Puglia:** orecchiette with turnip greens.
- **Sicily:** pasta alla norma, pasta with sardines.

Knowing these specialties will allow you to appreciate the richness of Italian culinary tradition and always choose the right recipe for every occasion.

ConclusionPasta is not just food: it is a universal language that unites flavors, cultures, and people. Now that you have a general overview of Italian pasta, you're ready to get your hands dirty and dive into the preparation of authentic and delicious recipes.In the next chapter, we will explore the essential tools to have in your kitchen to best prepare every dish. Get ready to become true pasta masters!

Summary of the 75 Recipes for Italian Pasta-Based First Courses

01 Spaghetti with Tomato and Basil02 Penne all'Arrabbiata03 Bucatini all'Amatriciana04 Pasta alla Puttanesca05 Linguine with Olive and Caper Sauce06 Spaghetti with Cherry Tomato Sauce07 Rigatoni with Tomato and Ricotta08 Penne with Fresh Tomato and Burrata09 Fusilli with Tomato and Bell Pepper Sauce10 Pasta with Tomato and Eggplant11 Classic Spaghetti Carbonara12 Vegetarian Carbonara

Pasta13 Rigatoni Carbonara with Zucchini14 Seafood Carbonara Spaghetti15 Fusilli Carbonara with Crispy Pancetta16 Classic Bucatini all'Amatriciana17 Pasta alla Gricia with Guanciale18 Rigatoni Gricia with Artichokes19 Fettuccine with Spicy Amatriciana Sauce20 Pasta alla Gricia with Fava Beans21 Trofie with Genovese Pesto22 Spaghetti with Arugula and Walnut Pesto23 Pasta with Pistachio Pesto24 Fusilli with Almond and Sundried Tomato Pesto25 Orecchiette with Basil and Pecorino Pesto26 Lasagna alla Bolognese27 Cannelloni Stuffed with Ricotta and Spinach28 Baked Pasta with Ragù and Béchamel29 Lasagna with Pesto30 Ziti Sicilian-Style Baked Pasta31 Tagliatelle with Meat Ragù32 Pappardelle with Wild Boar Ragù33 Fusilli with Vegetable Ragù34 Penne with Lentil Ragù35 Ravioli with Mushroom Ragù36 Tagliatelle with Butter and Sage37 Ravioli Stuffed with Ricotta and

Lemon38 Potato Gnocchi with Tomato Sauce39 Tagliolini with Truffle40 Agnolotti Stuffed with Meat in Roast Sauce41 Linguine allo Scoglio (Seafood Linguine)42 Spaghetti with Clams43 Tagliolini with Squid Ink44 Paccheri with Shrimp and Zucchini45 Pasta with Octopus Ragù46 Tagliatelle with Porcini Mushrooms47 Pasta with Black Truffle and Parmesan48 Fusilli with Gorgonzola and Walnuts49 Ravioli Stuffed with Potatoes and Fontina50 Spaghetti with Mushrooms and Pancetta51 Whole-Wheat Penne with Tomato and Basil52 Gluten-Free Fusilli with Zucchini Pesto53 Whole-Wheat Spaghetti with Tomato and Tuna Sauce54 Gluten-Free Pasta with Vegetable Ragù55 Whole-Wheat Linguine with Eggplant and Salted Ricotta56 Spaghetti with Lemon and Shrimp57 Penne with Avocado and Lime Cream58 Fusilli with Bell Pepper and Almond Sauce59 Tagliatelle with Pumpkin and Amaretti Sauce60 Pasta with Mint Pesto and Peas61 Orecchiette with Turnip Greens (Puglia)62 Pici with Wild Boar Ragù (Tuscany)63 Trenette with Pesto (Liguria)64 Spaghetti alla Norma (Sicily)65 Bigoli in Salsa (Veneto)66 Spaghetti with Fresh Tomato and Basil67 Pasta with Seasonal Vegetables and EVOO68 Penne with Zucchini, Lemon, and Mint69 Fusilli with Broccoli and Almond Cream70 Linguine with Cherry Tomato and Oregano Sauce71 Seafood Lasagna with Lemon Béchamel72 Ravioli Stuffed with Pumpkin and Mustard73 Tagliolini with Lobster and Saffron74 Fettuccine with White Duck Ragù75 Gnocchi with Castelmagno and Truffle

1. 01 **Spaghetti with Tomato and Basil**

Ingredients (for 4 people):
- 400 g of spaghetti
- 500 g of ripe tomatoes (San Marzano or cherry tomatoes)
- 2 garlic cloves
- 4 tablespoons of extra virgin olive oil
- A few fresh basil leaves

- Salt to taste
- Grated Parmesan (optional)

Preparation time: 10 minutesCooking time: 20 minutes

Preparation:

1. **Prepare the tomatoes**: Bring a pot of water to a boil. Blanch the tomatoes for about 1 minute, then drain and peel them with a knife. Dice the tomatoes.
2. **Prepare the sauce**: In a large pan, heat the olive oil with the whole, crushed garlic cloves. Sauté the garlic for 2-3 minutes until golden, then remove it.
3. **Cook the sauce**: Add the diced tomatoes, season with salt, and cook over medium heat for 15 minutes, stirring occasionally.
4. **Cook the pasta**: Bring a large pot of salted water to a boil and cook the spaghetti according to the package instructions (about 8-10 minutes).
5. **Toss the pasta**: Drain the spaghetti al dente and transfer them directly into the pan with the sauce. Add the torn basil leaves and stir for 1-2 minutes.
6. **Serve**: Plate the pasta and, if desired, sprinkle with grated Parmesan.

2. 02 **Penne all'Arrabbiata**

Ingredients (for 4 people):
- 400 g of penne rigate
- 400 g of peeled tomatoes
- 2 dried red chili peppers
- 2 garlic cloves
- 4 tablespoons of extra virgin olive oil
- Salt to taste
- Fresh chopped parsley (optional)

Preparation time: 5 minutesCooking time: 20 minutes

Preparation:

1. **Prepare the sauce:** Heat the oil in a large pan, add the crushed garlic and crumbled chili peppers. Sauté for 2 minutes, then remove the garlic.

2. **Cook the sauce:** Add the peeled tomatoes, mash them with a fork, season with salt, and cook over medium heat for about 15 minutes, stirring occasionally.

3. **Cook the pasta:** While the sauce cooks, bring a large pot of salted water to a boil and cook the penne for 10-12 minutes until al dente.

4.   **Combine pasta and sauce**: Drain the penne and transfer them to the pan with the sauce. Toss for 2 minutes to combine the flavors.

5.   Serve: Plate the pasta and, if desired, garnish with fresh chopped parsley.

03 Bucatini all'Amatriciana

Ingredients (for 4 people):
- 400 g of bucatini
- 150 g of guanciale
- 350 g of peeled tomatoes
- 50 g of grated Pecorino Romano
- 1 chili pepper (optional)
- Salt to taste

Preparation time: 5 minutesCooking time: 25 minutes

Preparation:

1.   Prepare the guanciale: Cut the guanciale into strips. Heat a pan without adding oil and cook the guanciale over low heat for 5-6 minutes until crispy. Remove and set aside.

2.   Prepare the sauce: In the fat rendered from the guanciale, add the peeled tomatoes and chili pepper. Cook over

medium heat for about 15 minutes, seasoning lightly with salt.

3. **Cook the pasta**: Boil the bucatini in a large pot of salted water for 8-10 minutes and drain al dente.

4. **Assemble the dish**: Combine the bucatini with the sauce, add the crispy guanciale, and toss for 2 minutes.

5. **Serve**: Finish with a generous sprinkle of grated Pecorino Romano and serve immediately.

4. 04 **Pasta alla Puttanesca**

Ingredients (for 4 people):
- 400 g of spaghetti
- 300 g of peeled tomatoes
- 100 g of pitted black olives
- 2 tablespoons of capers in salt
- 4 anchovy fillets in oil
- 2 garlic cloves
- 4 tablespoons of extra virgin olive oil
- Salt to taste
- Fresh chopped parsley (optional)

Preparation time: 10 minutesCooking time: 20 minutes

Preparation:

1.   **Prepare the ingredients**: Rinse the capers under running water to remove excess salt and slice the olives into rings.

2.   **Prepare the sauce**: Heat the olive oil in a pan, add the garlic and anchovies. Sauté over low heat until the anchovies dissolve.

3.   **Cook the sauce**: Add the peeled tomatoes, mash them with a fork, and mix in the olives and capers. Cook for 15 minutes over medium heat.

4.   **Cook the pasta**: Boil the spaghetti in salted water for 8-10 minutes.

5.   **Toss the pasta**: Drain the spaghetti and toss them in the pan with the sauce for 2 minutes.

6.   **Serve**: Plate the pasta and garnish with fresh parsley, if desired.

5.   05 **Linguine with Olive and Caper Sauce**

Ingredients (for 4 people):
- 400 g of linguine
- 300 g of ripe tomatoes
- 100 g of pitted black olives
- 2 tablespoons of capers in salt

- 2 garlic cloves
- 4 tablespoons of extra virgin olive oil
- Salt and pepper to taste
- Fresh parsley (optional)

Preparation time: 10 minutesCooking time: 20 minutes

Preparation:

1. **Prepare the tomatoes**: Blanch the tomatoes for 1 minute, peel them, remove the seeds, and chop them.
2. **Rinse the capers**: Rinse the capers under running water to remove excess salt.
3. **Prepare the sauce**: Heat the oil in a pan with the crushed garlic. When the garlic is golden, remove it. Add the tomatoes, olives, and capers. Cook over medium heat for about 15 minutes. Season with salt and pepper.
4. **Cook the linguine**: Boil the linguine in a large pot of salted water for 8-10 minutes.
5. **Assemble the dish**: Drain the linguine al dente and transfer them to the pan with the sauce. Toss for 2 minutes to combine the flavors.

6. **Serve**: Finish with fresh chopped parsley, if desired.

6. 06 **Spaghetti with Cherry Tomato Sauce**

Ingredients (for 4 people):
- 400 g of spaghetti
- 300 g of cherry tomatoes
- 2 garlic cloves
- 4 tablespoons of extra virgin olive oil
- Salt and pepper to taste
- Fresh basil to taste

Preparation time: 10 minutesCooking time: 15 minutes

Preparation:

1. **Prepare the cherry tomatoes**: Wash the cherry tomatoes and cut them in half.

2. **Prepare the sauce**: Heat the olive oil in a large pan with the crushed garlic. Add the cherry tomatoes and cook over medium heat for 10 minutes. Season with salt and pepper.

3. **Cook the spaghetti**: Cook the spaghetti in boiling salted water for about 8 minutes.

4. **Assemble the dish**: Drain the spaghetti and toss them directly in the pan with the sauce for 2 minutes.
5. **Serve**: Garnish with fresh basil leaves and serve.

7. 07 **Rigatoni with Tomato and Ricotta**

Ingredients (for 4 people):
- 400 g of rigatoni
- 300 g of peeled tomatoes
- 150 g of fresh ricotta
- 2 tablespoons of extra virgin olive oil
- Salt and pepper to taste
- Fresh basil to taste

Preparation time: 10 minutesCooking time: 20 minutes

Preparation:

1. **Prepare the sauce**: Blend the peeled tomatoes to create a smooth puree. Heat the olive oil in a pan, add the puree, and cook over medium heat for 10 minutes. Season with salt and pepper.
2. **Cook the rigatoni**: Boil the rigatoni in salted water for 12 minutes or until al dente.

3.   **Assemble the dish**: Drain the rigatoni, add them to the sauce, and mix in the ricotta. Stir gently until creamy.
4.   **Serve**: Garnish with fresh basil leaves and serve immediately.

8.   08 **Penne with Fresh Tomato and Burrata**

Ingredients (for 4 people):
- 400 g of penne rigate
- 400 g of fresh tomatoes
- 200 g of burrata
- 3 tablespoons of extra virgin olive oil
- Salt and pepper to taste
- Fresh basil to taste

Preparation time: 10 minutesCooking time: 15 minutes
Preparation:
1.   **Prepare the tomatoes**: Blanch the tomatoes for 1 minute, peel them, and chop them into pieces.
2.   **Prepare the sauce**: Heat the olive oil in a pan, add the tomatoes, and cook for 10 minutes. Season with salt and pepper.

3.   **Cook the penne**: Boil the pasta in abundant salted water for about 10 minutes.

4.   **Assemble the dish**: Drain the pasta, mix it with the sauce, and stir well. Plate the dish and top each serving with pieces of burrata.

5.   **Decorate**: Finish with fresh basil leaves and serve.

9.   09 **Fusilli with Tomato and Bell Pepper Sauce**

Ingredients (for 4 people):
*   400 g of fusilli
*   1 red bell pepper
*   300 g of peeled tomatoes
*   2 tablespoons of extra virgin olive oil
*   1 small onion
*   Salt and pepper to taste

Preparation time: 15 minutesCooking time: 20 minutes

Preparation:

1.   **Roast the bell pepper**: Roast the bell pepper in the oven at 200°C for 15 minutes. Once cooled, peel and cut it into pieces.

2.   **Prepare the sauce**: Finely chop the onion and sauté it in a pan with olive oil. Add the peeled tomatoes and roasted bell pepper, then blend everything into a smooth cream. Season with salt and pepper.

3.   **Cook the fusilli**: Cook the pasta al dente in salted water for 10-12 minutes.

4.   **Assemble the dish**: Drain the fusilli, toss them with the sauce, and mix well.

5.   **Serve**: Serve hot, optionally with a sprinkle of grated Parmesan.

10. 10 Pasta with Tomato and Eggplant

Ingredients (for 4 people):
- 400 g of short pasta (e.g., mezze maniche)
- 1 large eggplant
- 300 g of peeled tomatoes
- 4 tablespoons of extra virgin olive oil
- Salt and pepper to taste
- Fresh basil

Preparation time: 10 minutesCooking time: 25 minutes

Preparation:

1.   **Prepare the eggplant**: Cut the eggplant into cubes and fry them in abundant oil until golden. Drain on paper towels.
2.   **Prepare the sauce**: In a pan, heat the olive oil, add the peeled and crushed tomatoes, and cook for 15 minutes. Season with salt and pepper.
3.   **Cook the pasta**: Boil the pasta in salted water for 10 minutes.
4.   **Assemble the dish**: Combine the pasta with the sauce, add the eggplant, and stir gently.
5.   **Serve**: Garnish with fresh basil and serve hot.

11.11 Classic Spaghetti Carbonara

Ingredients (for 4 people):
- 400 g of spaghetti
- 150 g of guanciale
- 3 eggs (2 whole and 1 yolk)
- 80 g of grated Pecorino Romano
- Freshly ground black pepper to taste
- Salt to taste

Preparation time: 10 minutesCooking time: 15 minutes
Preparation:

1.   **Prepare the guanciale**: Cut the guanciale into strips. In a pan without oil, sauté it over low heat for 5-7 minutes until crispy. Turn off the heat and set it aside.
2.   **Prepare the egg mixture**: In a bowl, beat the eggs with Pecorino and a generous grind of black pepper. Mix until smooth.
3.   **Cook the pasta**: Cook the spaghetti in boiling salted water for about 8-10 minutes, draining it al dente.
4.   **Assemble the dish**: Transfer the spaghetti directly to the pan with the guanciale. Off the heat, pour in the egg mixture and mix quickly to combine. The heat from the pasta will gently cook the eggs, creating a creamy sauce.
5.   **Serve**: Plate the pasta, top with grated Pecorino, and a sprinkle of black pepper.

12.12 Vegetarian Carbonara Pasta

Ingredients (for 4 people):
- 400 g of penne rigate
- 2 medium zucchinis
- 3 eggs (2 whole and 1 yolk)

- 80 g of grated Pecorino Romano or Parmesan
- 2 tablespoons of extra virgin olive oil
- Freshly ground black pepper to taste
- Salt to taste

Preparation time: 15 minutesCooking time: 20 minutes

Preparation:

1. **Prepare the zucchinis**: Wash the zucchinis, cut them into cubes, and sauté them in a pan with olive oil for 5-7 minutes until golden but still firm.
2. **Prepare the egg mixture**: Beat the eggs in a bowl with grated cheese, black pepper, and a pinch of salt.
3. **Cook the pasta**: Boil the penne in salted water for about 10-12 minutes.
4. **Assemble the dish**: Drain the pasta al dente, add it to the pan with the zucchinis, and mix. Off the heat, add the egg mixture and stir quickly.
5. **Serve**: Plate the pasta, top with more black pepper and grated cheese, and serve immediately.

13. 13 Rigatoni Carbonara with Zucchini

Ingredients (for 4 people):
- 400 g of rigatoni
- 3 medium zucchinis
- 3 eggs (2 whole and 1 yolk)
- 100 g of grated Pecorino Romano
- 2 tablespoons of extra virgin olive oil
- Freshly ground black pepper to taste
- Salt to taste

Preparation time: 15 minutesCooking time: 20 minutes

Preparation:

1. **Prepare the zucchinis**: Cut the zucchinis into slices and sauté them in a pan with oil for 5-7 minutes until golden. Lightly salt and set aside.

2. **Prepare the egg mixture**: Beat the eggs with Pecorino and black pepper until smooth.

3. **Cook the pasta**: Boil the rigatoni in salted water for about 10 minutes.

4. **Assemble the dish**: Drain the pasta al dente, transfer it to the pan with the zucchinis, and add the egg mixture off the heat. Stir quickly to avoid scrambling the eggs.

5. **Serve**: Top with a sprinkle of Pecorino and black pepper and serve hot.

14.14 **Seafood Carbonara Spaghetti**

Ingredients (for 4 people):
- 400 g of spaghetti
- 200 g of peeled shrimp
- 2 eggs (1 whole and 1 yolk)
- 50 g of grated Pecorino Romano
- 2 tablespoons of extra virgin olive oil
- Freshly ground black pepper to taste
- Salt to taste

Preparation time: 15 minutesCooking time: 20 minutes
Preparation:
1. **Sauté the shrimp**: Heat the oil in a pan and sauté the shrimp for 3-4 minutes until golden. Set them aside.
2. **Prepare the egg mixture**: In a bowl, beat the eggs with Pecorino and a generous grind of black pepper.
3. **Cook the pasta**: Cook the spaghetti in salted water for 8-10 minutes, draining it al dente.
4. **Assemble the dish**: Transfer the spaghetti to the pan with the shrimp, turn off the heat, and add the egg mixture. Mix thoroughly until creamy.

5.   **Serve**: Garnish with black pepper and a drizzle of raw olive oil if desired.

15.15 Fusilli Carbonara with Crispy Pancetta

Ingredients (for 4 people):
*   400 g of fusilli
*   150 g of smoked pancetta
*   3 eggs (2 whole and 1 yolk)
*   80 g of grated Parmesan or Pecorino Romano
*   Freshly ground black pepper to taste
*   Salt to taste

Preparation time: 10 minutesCooking time: 15 minutes

Preparation:

1.   **Prepare the pancetta**: Cut the pancetta into cubes. Sauté it in a pan without oil for 5-6 minutes until crispy.
2.   **Prepare the egg mixture**: Beat the eggs with grated cheese and a generous grind of black pepper.
3.   **Cook the pasta**: Boil the fusilli in salted water for 10-12 minutes and drain al dente.

4.   **Assemble the dish**: Add the fusilli to the pan with the pancetta. Off the heat, pour in the egg mixture and stir quickly.
5.   **Serve**: Top with more black pepper and serve immediately.

16. 16 Classic Bucatini all'Amatriciana

Ingredients (for 4 people):
- 400 g of bucatini
- 150 g of guanciale
- 400 g of peeled tomatoes
- 50 g of grated Pecorino Romano
- 1 chili pepper (optional)
- Salt to taste

Preparation time: 10 minutesCooking time: 25 minutes
Preparation:
1.   **Prepare the guanciale**: Cut the guanciale into strips. Sauté it in a pan without oil over low heat for 5-6 minutes until crispy. Set the guanciale aside and keep the rendered fat.
2.   **Prepare the sauce**: In the same pan, add the peeled tomatoes, crushed with a fork, and the chili pepper (if desired).

Cook over medium heat for 15 minutes, seasoning lightly with salt.

3. **Cook the bucatini**: Boil a large pot of salted water and cook the bucatini for 8-10 minutes.

4. **Assemble the dish**: Drain the bucatini al dente, transfer them to the pan with the sauce, and add the crispy guanciale. Mix well.

5. **Serve**: Top with grated Pecorino Romano and serve hot.

17.17 Pasta alla Gricia with Guanciale

Ingredients (for 4 people):
- 400 g of rigatoni
- 150 g of guanciale
- 60 g of grated Pecorino Romano
- Freshly ground black pepper to taste
- Salt to taste

Preparation time: 5 minutesCooking time: 20 minutes

Preparation:

1. **Prepare the guanciale**: Cut the guanciale into strips and sauté it in a pan without oil over medium heat for 5-7 minutes until crispy. Keep the rendered fat.

2.   **Cook the pasta**: Cook the rigatoni in abundant salted water for about 10 minutes.

3.   **Assemble the dish**: Drain the pasta al dente, reserving a cup of cooking water. Toss the rigatoni in the pan with the guanciale and its fat, adding a bit of cooking water to create a creamy texture.

4.   **Serve**: Plate the pasta, sprinkle generously with Pecorino and black pepper, and serve hot.

18.18 Rigatoni Gricia with Artichokes

Ingredients (for 4 people):
- 400 g of rigatoni
- 2 artichokes
- 150 g of guanciale
- 60 g of grated Pecorino Romano
- 2 tablespoons of extra virgin olive oil
- Lemon juice to taste
- Freshly ground black pepper to taste
- Salt to taste

Preparation time: 15 minutesCooking time: 25 minutes

Preparation:

1.   **Prepare the artichokes**: Clean the artichokes, removing the tough outer leaves and inner choke. Slice them thinly and soak them in water with lemon juice to prevent browning.

2.   **Prepare the guanciale**: Sauté the guanciale in a pan without oil until crispy. Add the drained artichokes and cook for 8-10 minutes until tender.

3.   **Cook the pasta**: Boil the rigatoni in salted water for about 10 minutes.

4.   **Assemble the dish**: Drain the pasta al dente and transfer it to the pan with the guanciale and artichokes. Add a ladle of cooking water and toss to combine.

5.   **Serve**: Sprinkle with Pecorino and black pepper and serve immediately.

19. 19 Spicy Amatriciana Fettuccine

Ingredients (for 4 people):
- 400 g of fresh fettuccine
- 150 g of guanciale
- 400 g of peeled tomatoes
- 1 red chili pepper
- 50 g of grated Pecorino Romano
- 2 tablespoons of extra virgin olive oil

- Salt to taste

Preparation time: 10 minutesCooking time: 20 minutes

Preparation:

1. **Prepare the guanciale**: Sauté the guanciale, cut into strips, in a pan without oil for 5-6 minutes until crispy.
2. **Prepare the sauce**: Add the crushed peeled tomatoes and diced chili pepper to the pan. Cook for 10-15 minutes over medium heat, seasoning with salt.
3. **Cook the pasta**: Boil the fettuccine in salted water for 4-5 minutes (if fresh).
4. **Assemble the dish**: Drain the fettuccine and toss them in the pan with the sauce. Add a ladle of cooking water if needed to combine everything well.
5. **Serve**: Top with grated Pecorino Romano and serve immediately.

20.20 Pasta alla Gricia with Fava Beans

Ingredients (for 4 people):

- 400 g of rigatoni
- 150 g of guanciale
- 100 g of fresh fava beans (or frozen)
- 60 g of grated Pecorino Romano

- 1 tablespoon of extra virgin olive oil
- Freshly ground black pepper to taste
- Salt to taste

Preparation time: 10 minutesCooking time: 25 minutes

Preparation:

1. **Prepare the fava beans**: Blanch the fava beans in boiling water for 2 minutes, then cool them under running water and remove the outer skins.

2. **Prepare the guanciale**: Sauté the guanciale, cut into strips, in a pan without oil until crispy. Add the fava beans and cook for 5 minutes over low heat.

3. **Cook the pasta**: Cook the rigatoni in abundant salted water for 10 minutes.

4. **Assemble the dish**: Drain the rigatoni al dente, transfer them to the pan with the guanciale and fava beans, and add a ladle of cooking water. Toss to combine the flavors.

5. **Serve**: Plate the pasta and finish with grated Pecorino and black pepper.

21.21 Trofie with Genovese Pesto

Ingredients (for 4 people):

- 400 g of fresh trofie
- 50 g of fresh basil
- 30 g of pine nuts
- 2 garlic cloves
- 50 g of grated Parmesan cheese
- 30 g of grated Pecorino Sardo cheese
- 100 ml of extra virgin olive oil
- Coarse salt to taste

Preparation time: 15 minutesCooking time: 10 minutes

Preparation:

1. **Prepare the pesto**: In a mortar, crush the garlic with a pinch of coarse salt. Add the basil leaves and gently pound. Incorporate the pine nuts, followed by the cheeses, and slowly add the olive oil. Continue pounding until you obtain a smooth paste. Alternatively, you can use a blender, but pulse gently to avoid overheating the pesto.

2. **Cook the trofie**: Bring a pot of salted water to a boil and cook the trofie for 8-10 minutes.

3. **Season the pasta**: Drain the trofie, reserving a ladle of cooking water. Toss

the pasta with the pesto, adding the cooking water to blend the sauce.
4. **Serve**: Plate and serve immediately, garnishing with fresh basil leaves.

22.22 Spaghetti with Arugula and Walnut Pesto

Ingredients (for 4 people):
- 400 g of spaghetti
- 100 g of fresh arugula
- 50 g of shelled walnuts
- 1 garlic clove
- 50 g of grated Parmesan cheese
- 80 ml of extra virgin olive oil
- Salt and pepper to taste

Preparation time: 10 minutesCooking time: 10 minutes
Preparation:
1. **Prepare the pesto**: Blend the arugula, walnuts, garlic, Parmesan, and olive oil until smooth. Season with salt and pepper.
2. **Cook the spaghetti**: Boil the spaghetti in salted water for about 8 minutes, draining it al dente.

3.   **Assemble the dish**: Toss the spaghetti with the arugula pesto, adding a ladle of cooking water to make the sauce creamier.

4.   **Serve**: Garnish with walnut pieces and a sprinkle of Parmesan cheese.

23.23 Pasta with Pistachio Pesto

Ingredients (for 4 people):
- 400 g of short pasta (e.g., penne or fusilli)
- 100 g of shelled, unsalted pistachios
- 50 g of grated Parmesan cheese
- 80 ml of extra virgin olive oil
- 1 garlic clove (optional)
- Salt and pepper to taste

Preparation time: 10 minutesCooking time: 10 minutes

Preparation:

1.   **Prepare the pistachio pesto**: Blend the pistachios with Parmesan, olive oil, and garlic (if desired). Add salt and pepper and blend until smooth.

2.   **Cook the pasta**: Boil the pasta in salted water and drain it al dente.

3.   **Season the pasta**: Mix the pasta with the pistachio pesto, adding some cooking water to achieve a creamy texture.

4.   **Serve**: Garnish with chopped pistachios and serve immediately.

24.24 **Fusilli with Almond and Sundried Tomato Pesto**

Ingredients (for 4 people):
- 400 g of fusilli
- 80 g of shelled almonds
- 50 g of sundried tomatoes in oil
- 30 g of grated Parmesan cheese
- 50 ml of extra virgin olive oil
- 1 garlic clove
- Salt and pepper to taste

Preparation time: 10 minutesCooking time: 12 minutes

Preparation:

1.   **Prepare the pesto**: Blend the almonds, sundried tomatoes, Parmesan, garlic, and olive oil into a thick paste. Adjust with salt and pepper to taste.

2.   **Cook the fusilli**: Boil the pasta in salted water for about 10-12 minutes and drain al dente.

3.   **Season the pasta**: Mix the fusilli with the pesto, adding a ladle of cooking water to combine.

4.   **Serve**: Decorate with chopped almonds and a drizzle of raw olive oil.

25.25 Orecchiette with Basil and Pecorino Pesto

Ingredients (for 4 people):
- 400 g of orecchiette
- 50 g of fresh basil
- 30 g of pine nuts
- 50 g of grated Pecorino Romano
- 80 ml of extra virgin olive oil
- 1 garlic clove
- Coarse salt to taste

Preparation time: 15 minutesCooking time: 12 minutes

Preparation:

1.   **Prepare the pesto**: In a mortar, crush the garlic with a pinch of coarse salt. Add the basil leaves and pine nuts,

pounding to combine. Gradually mix in the Pecorino and olive oil until smooth.

2. **Cook the orecchiette**: Boil the pasta in abundant salted water for about 10-12 minutes.

3. **Season the pasta**: Drain the orecchiette and mix them with the pesto. Add a bit of cooking water to blend the sauce better.

4. **Serve**: Plate and garnish with fresh basil leaves and grated Pecorino.

26.26 Lasagna Bolognese

Ingredients (for 6 people):
- 500 g of fresh egg lasagna sheets
- 500 g of Bolognese ragù (prepared beforehand)
- 500 ml of béchamel sauce
- 150 g of grated Parmesan cheese
- Butter to taste

Preparation time: 30 minutesCooking time: 30-40 minutes

Preparation:

1. **Prepare the ingredients**: Prepare the ragù and béchamel sauce if not already done. Preheat the oven to 180°C.

2.   **Assemble the lasagna**: In a buttered baking dish, spread a layer of ragù, then cover with a layer of lasagna sheets. Add another layer of ragù, a layer of béchamel, and a sprinkle of Parmesan. Repeat until all the ingredients are used, finishing with a layer of béchamel and Parmesan.

3.   **Bake**: Bake the lasagna for 30-40 minutes, until the surface is golden brown.

4.   **Serve**: Let the lasagna rest for 10 minutes before serving.

27.27 Cannelloni Stuffed with Ricotta and Spinach

Ingredients (for 4 people):
- 250 g of dry cannelloni
- 500 g of fresh spinach
- 300 g of ricotta
- 100 g of grated Parmesan cheese
- 500 ml of béchamel sauce
- 400 g of tomato sauce
- 1 garlic clove
- Extra virgin olive oil to taste
- Nutmeg to taste

- Salt and pepper to taste

Preparation time: 40 minutesCooking time: 30 minutes

Preparation:

1. **Prepare the filling**: Blanch the spinach, drain, and chop finely. Mix with ricotta, half the Parmesan, a pinch of nutmeg, salt, and pepper.
2. **Fill the cannelloni**: Use a piping bag or a small spoon to fill the cannelloni with the ricotta and spinach mixture.
3. **Prepare the sauce**: In a pan, heat the oil with the garlic, add the tomato sauce, season with salt, and cook for 10 minutes.
4. **Assemble the dish**: In a baking dish, spread a layer of tomato sauce, arrange the cannelloni on top, and cover with the remaining tomato sauce and béchamel. Sprinkle with Parmesan.
5. **Bake**: Bake at 180°C for 30 minutes. Serve hot.

28.28 Baked Pasta with Ragù and Béchamel

Ingredients (for 6 people):

- 400 g of short pasta (e.g., rigatoni or penne)
- 500 g of meat ragù
- 500 ml of béchamel sauce
- 200 g of diced mozzarella
- 150 g of grated Parmesan cheese
- Butter to taste

Preparation time: 20 minutesCooking time: 30 minutes

Preparation:

1. **Prepare the ingredients**: Prepare the ragù and béchamel if not already done. Cook the pasta in abundant salted water, draining it very al dente.
2. **Assemble the dish**: Mix the pasta with the ragù and half the béchamel. In a buttered baking dish, layer the pasta, alternating with mozzarella and Parmesan. Finish with a layer of béchamel and Parmesan.
3. **Bake**: Bake at 200°C for 30 minutes, until golden.
4. **Serve**: Let it cool for 5 minutes before serving.

29.29 Lasagna with Pesto

Ingredients (for 6 people):
- 500 g of fresh egg lasagna sheets
- 300 g of Genovese pesto
- 500 ml of béchamel sauce
- 150 g of grated Parmesan cheese
- Butter to taste

Preparation time: 25 minutesCooking time: 30 minutes

Preparation:

1. **Prepare the ingredients**: Mix the pesto with half the béchamel to create a creamy sauce. Preheat the oven to 180°C.

2. **Assemble the lasagna**: In a buttered baking dish, spread a layer of pesto sauce, then a layer of lasagna sheets. Alternate layers until all ingredients are used, finishing with a layer of sauce and Parmesan.

3. **Bake**: Bake for 30 minutes.

4. **Serve**: Let rest for 10 minutes before serving.

30.30 Baked Ziti Sicilian Style

Ingredients (for 4 people):
- 400 g of ziti

- 1 large eggplant
- 400 g of tomato sauce
- 200 g of grated salted ricotta
- 150 g of diced mozzarella
- 1 garlic clove
- Extra virgin olive oil to taste
- Fresh basil to taste
- Salt to taste

Preparation time: 20 minutesCooking time: 40 minutes

Preparation:

1. **Prepare the eggplants**: Cut the eggplant into cubes and fry them in abundant hot oil. Drain on paper towels.

2. **Prepare the sauce**: In a pan, sauté the garlic with a drizzle of oil, add the tomato sauce, season with salt, and cook for 10 minutes. Add basil at the end.

3. **Cook the ziti**: Break the ziti in half and boil them in salted water for half the time indicated on the package.

4. **Assemble the dish**: Mix the ziti with half the sauce, the eggplants, half the ricotta, and mozzarella. Place everything in a baking dish, covering with the remaining sauce and ricotta.

5. **Bake**: Bake at 180°C for 30 minutes. Serve hot.

31.31 Tagliatelle with Meat Ragù

Ingredients (for 4 people):
- 400 g of fresh tagliatelle
- 300 g of mixed ground meat (beef and pork)
- 200 g of tomato purée
- 1 carrot
- 1 celery stalk
- 1 small onion
- 1 glass of red wine
- 3 tablespoons of extra virgin olive oil
- 1 bay leaf
- Salt and pepper to taste
- Grated Parmesan cheese to taste

Preparation time: 15 minutesCooking time: 1 hour 30 minutes

Preparation:

1. **Prepare the soffritto**: Finely chop the carrot, celery, and onion. Heat the oil in a saucepan and sauté the mixture for 5 minutes.

2.   **Add the meat**: Add the ground meat to the soffritto and cook for 10 minutes, breaking it up with a wooden spoon.

3.   **Deglaze with wine**: Pour in the red wine and let it evaporate completely.

4.   **Prepare the ragù**: Add the tomato purée, bay leaf, a pinch of salt, and pepper. Cover and cook on low heat for at least 1 hour, stirring occasionally.

5.   **Cook the tagliatelle**: Bring a pot of salted water to a boil, cook the tagliatelle for 2-3 minutes (if fresh), and drain.

6.   **Assemble the dish**: Toss the tagliatelle with the ragù and finish with grated Parmesan.

32. 32 Pappardelle with Wild Boar Ragù

Ingredients (for 4 people):
- 400 g of fresh pappardelle
- 300 g of wild boar meat
- 1 onion
- 1 carrot
- 1 celery stalk
- 2 glasses of red wine
- 200 g of tomato purée

- 2 sprigs of rosemary
- 1 bay leaf
- Extra virgin olive oil to taste
- Salt and pepper to taste

Preparation time: 20 minutesCooking time: 2 hours 30 minutes

Preparation:

1. **Marinate the wild boar**: Cut the meat into cubes and marinate it with red wine, rosemary, and bay leaf for at least 12 hours in the refrigerator.

2. **Prepare the soffritto**: Finely chop the onion, carrot, and celery. Heat the oil in a saucepan and sauté the soffritto for 5 minutes.

3. **Sear the wild boar**: Drain the wild boar from the marinade, pat it dry, and brown it in the soffritto.

4. **Prepare the ragù**: Add the marinade wine, let it evaporate, then add the tomato purée, bay leaf, rosemary, salt, and pepper. Cover and simmer on low heat for at least 2 hours.

5. **Cook the pappardelle**: Cook the fresh pasta for 2-3 minutes, drain, and mix with the ragù.

6.   **Serve**: Drizzle with a bit of raw olive oil and serve hot.

33. 33 Fusilli with Vegetable Ragù

Ingredients (for 4 people):
- 400 g of fusilli
- 1 zucchini
- 1 small eggplant
- 1 carrot
- 1 red bell pepper
- 200 g of tomato purée
- 1 small onion
- 2 tablespoons of extra virgin olive oil
- Salt and pepper to taste
- Fresh basil to taste

Preparation time: 15 minutesCooking time: 40 minutes

Preparation:

1.   **Prepare the vegetables**: Wash and dice the zucchini, eggplant, carrot, and bell pepper. Finely chop the onion.

2.   **Sauté the vegetables**: Heat the oil in a large pan and sauté the onion. Add the vegetables and cook for 15 minutes, stirring often.

3. **Prepare the ragù**: Add the tomato purée, season with salt and pepper, and cook on low heat for 20 minutes, stirring occasionally.

4. **Cook the fusilli**: Boil a pot of salted water, cook the fusilli for 10-12 minutes, and drain them al dente.

5. **Assemble the dish**: Toss the fusilli with the vegetable ragù, add fresh basil, and serve.

34. 34 **Penne with Lentil Ragù**

Ingredients (for 4 people):
- 400 g of penne rigate
- 150 g of dried lentils
- 1 carrot
- 1 celery stalk
- 1 small onion
- 200 g of tomato purée
- 1 glass of vegetable broth
- 2 tablespoons of extra virgin olive oil
- Salt and pepper to taste
- Grated Parmesan cheese (optional)

Preparation time: 10 minutesCooking time: 1 hour
Preparation:

1.   **Prepare the soffritto**: Finely chop the carrot, celery, and onion. Heat the oil in a saucepan and sauté the mixture for 5 minutes.

2.   **Add the lentils**: Rinse the lentils, add them to the soffritto, and sauté for a few minutes.

3.   **Prepare the ragù**: Add the tomato purée and vegetable broth. Simmer on low heat for 40-50 minutes, stirring occasionally. Season with salt and pepper.

4.   **Cook the pasta**: Boil the penne in salted water for about 10 minutes.

5.   **Assemble the dish**: Toss the pasta with the lentil ragù and, if desired, top with grated Parmesan.

35.35 Ravioli with Mushroom Ragù

Ingredients (for 4 people):
*   500 g of ricotta and spinach-filled ravioli
*   300 g of mixed mushrooms (porcini, champignon, etc.)
*   1 garlic clove
*   200 ml of fresh cream

- 2 tablespoons of extra virgin olive oil
- Fresh parsley to taste
- Salt and pepper to taste

Preparation time: 15 minutesCooking time: 20 minutes

Preparation:

1. **Prepare the mushrooms**: Clean and slice the mushrooms. Heat the oil in a pan with the garlic, add the mushrooms, and cook over medium heat for 10 minutes. Season with salt and pepper.

2. **Prepare the ragù**: Add the cream to the mushrooms and cook for another 5 minutes over low heat until a creamy sauce forms.

3. **Cook the ravioli**: Boil the ravioli in salted water for 3-4 minutes.

4. **Assemble the dish**: Drain the ravioli, toss them with the mushroom ragù, and finish with freshly chopped parsley.

36. 36 Tagliatelle with Butter and Sage

Ingredients (for 4 people):
- 400 g of fresh tagliatelle
- 80 g of butter
- 8 fresh sage leaves

- 50 g of grated Parmesan cheese
- Salt to taste

Preparation time: 5 minutesCooking time: 5 minutes

Preparation:

1. **Prepare the sauce**: In a large pan, melt the butter over low heat with the sage leaves. Let it infuse for 2-3 minutes, ensuring the butter does not burn.
2. **Cook the tagliatelle**: Bring a pot of salted water to a boil, cook the fresh tagliatelle for 2-3 minutes, and drain.
3. **Combine the dish**: Add the tagliatelle to the pan with the butter and sage. Toss for 1 minute to combine the flavors.
4. **Serve**: Plate the pasta and top with grated Parmesan cheese.

37. 37 Ravioli Stuffed with Ricotta and Lemon

Ingredients (for 4 people):
- 500 g of ricotta and lemon-filled ravioli
- 80 g of butter
- Zest of 1 organic lemon, grated
- 50 g of grated Parmesan cheese
- Freshly ground black pepper to taste

- Salt to taste

Preparation time: 5 minutesCooking time: 5 minutes

Preparation:

1. **Prepare the sauce**: In a pan, melt the butter over low heat. Add the grated lemon zest and a pinch of black pepper.
2. **Cook the ravioli**: Cook the ravioli in boiling salted water for 3-4 minutes and gently drain.
3. **Combine the dish**: Toss the ravioli gently in the pan with the sauce for 1 minute.
4. **Serve**: Top with grated Parmesan and serve immediately.

38. 38 Potato Gnocchi with Tomato Sauce

Ingredients (for 4 people):
- 500 g of potato gnocchi
- 400 g of tomato purée
- 2 garlic cloves
- 3 tablespoons of extra virgin olive oil
- Fresh basil to taste
- Salt to taste
- Grated Parmesan cheese to taste

Preparation time: 10 minutesCooking time: 15 minutes

Preparation:

1. **Prepare the sauce**: In a pan, heat the olive oil and sauté the whole garlic cloves. Add the tomato purée, season with salt, and simmer on low heat for 10-15 minutes. Add fresh basil leaves at the end of cooking.
2. **Cook the gnocchi**: Bring a pot of salted water to a boil and cook the gnocchi. When they float to the surface, gently drain them.
3. **Combine the dish**: Toss the gnocchi with the tomato sauce.
4. **Serve**: Plate and top with grated Parmesan cheese and fresh basil.

39. 39 Tagliolini with Truffle

Ingredients (for 4 people):
- 400 g of fresh tagliolini
- 50 g of fresh black truffle
- 80 g of butter
- 50 g of grated Parmesan cheese
- Salt to taste

Preparation time: 5 minutesCooking time: 5 minutes

Preparation:

1. **Prepare the sauce**: In a pan, melt the butter over low heat. Grate half of the truffle into the butter and let it infuse for 1-2 minutes.
2. **Cook the tagliolini**: Cook the fresh tagliolini in salted boiling water for 2-3 minutes.
3. **Combine the dish**: Drain the tagliolini and add them to the pan with the truffle butter. Toss for 1 minute.
4. **Serve**: Plate the pasta and garnish with thin slices of fresh truffle and grated Parmesan cheese.

40.40 Agnolotti Stuffed with Meat in Roast Sauce

Ingredients (for 4 people):
- 500 g of meat-filled agnolotti
- 300 ml of roast sauce (from the cooking juices of roast meat)
- 1 knob of butter
- Grated Parmesan cheese to taste
- Freshly ground black pepper to taste

Preparation time: 10 minutesCooking time: 5 minutes
Preparation:
1. **Prepare the roast sauce**: Heat the meat's cooking juices in a pan. If needed, add a knob of butter to make it creamier.
2. **Cook the agnolotti**: Cook the agnolotti in salted boiling water for 3-4 minutes and gently drain.
3. **Combine the dish**: Toss the agnolotti in the pan with the roast sauce for 1 minute.
4. **Serve**: Plate and finish with grated Parmesan and a grind of black pepper.

41.41 Linguine allo Scoglio

Ingredients (for 4 people):
- 400 g of linguine
- 200 g of mussels
- 200 g of clams
- 200 g of peeled shrimp
- 200 g of calamari, sliced into rings
- 300 g of cherry tomatoes
- 2 garlic cloves
- 4 tablespoons of extra virgin olive oil
- 1 glass of white wine

- Fresh parsley, chopped, to taste
- Salt and pepper to taste

Preparation time: 20 minutesCooking time: 20 minutes

Preparation:

1. **Clean the seafood**: Thoroughly clean the mussels and clams, removing any impurities. Rinse the shrimp and calamari.
2. **Prepare the sauce**: In a large pan, heat the oil with the garlic. Add the mussels and clams, deglaze with white wine, and cover. Cook for 5 minutes until the shells open. Remove the shellfish from the shells (leaving a few for decoration) and strain the cooking liquid.
3. **Cook the calamari and shrimp**: In the same pan, add the calamari and cook for 3 minutes. Add the halved cherry tomatoes, shrimp, and the strained liquid. Cook for another 5 minutes.
4. **Cook the linguine**: Boil the linguine in salted water and drain al dente.
5. **Assemble the dish**: Toss the linguine with the seafood sauce and shellfish. Sauté for 2 minutes.

6. **Serve**: Garnish with chopped parsley and serve.

42.42 Spaghetti alle Vongole Veraci

Ingredients (for 4 people):
- 400 g of spaghetti
- 1 kg of veracious clams
- 2 garlic cloves
- 4 tablespoons of extra virgin olive oil
- 1 glass of white wine
- Fresh parsley, chopped, to taste
- Salt and pepper to taste

Preparation time: 15 minutesCooking time: 15 minutes

Preparation:

1. **Purge the clams**: Soak the clams in salted water for at least 1 hour to remove sand. Rinse thoroughly.

2. **Cook the clams**: Heat the oil with garlic in a pan. Add the clams, deglaze with white wine, and cover. Cook for 5 minutes until they open. Strain the cooking liquid and set it aside.

3. **Prepare the sauce**: Remove some of the clams from their shells. Add the strained liquid to the pan and heat for 2 minutes.

4. **Cook the spaghetti**: Cook the spaghetti in salted water and drain al dente.

5. **Assemble the dish**: Toss the spaghetti with the sauce and clams. Garnish with fresh parsley.

6. **Serve**: Plate and decorate with a few clams in their shells.

43.43 Tagliolini al Nero di Seppia

Ingredients (for 4 people):
- 400 g of fresh squid ink tagliolini
- 300 g of calamari, sliced into rings
- 200 g of cherry tomatoes
- 1 garlic clove
- 1 chili pepper (optional)
- 4 tablespoons of extra virgin olive oil
- Fresh parsley, chopped, to taste
- Salt and pepper to taste

Preparation time: 10 minutesCooking time: 15 minutes

Preparation:

1. **Prepare the sauce**: Heat the oil in a pan with garlic and chili pepper. Add the calamari and cook for 5 minutes. Add the halved cherry tomatoes and cook for

another 5 minutes. Season with salt and pepper.

2. **Cook the tagliolini:** Cook the tagliolini in salted boiling water for 2-3 minutes.

3. **Assemble the dish:** Drain the tagliolini and toss them in the pan with the sauce for 2 minutes.

4. **Serve:** Plate the dish and top with fresh parsley.

44. 44 Paccheri with Shrimp and Zucchini

Ingredients (for 4 people):
- 400 g of paccheri
- 300 g of peeled shrimp
- 2 medium zucchinis
- 1 garlic clove
- 4 tablespoons of extra virgin olive oil
- 1 glass of white wine
- Salt and pepper to taste
- Fresh parsley, chopped, to taste

Preparation time: 10 minutesCooking time: 15 minutes

Preparation:

1. **Prepare the zucchinis:** Slice the zucchinis into thin rounds. Heat the oil

with garlic in a pan and sauté the zucchinis for 5 minutes.

2. **Cook the shrimp**: Add the shrimp to the pan, deglaze with white wine, and cook for 5 minutes. Season with salt and pepper.

3. **Cook the paccheri**: Cook the paccheri in salted water for about 10 minutes, draining al dente.

4. **Assemble the dish**: Toss the paccheri with the shrimp and zucchini sauce.

5. **Serve**: Garnish with chopped parsley and serve hot.

45.45 Pasta with Octopus Ragù

Ingredients (for 4 people):
- 400 g of short pasta (e.g., fusilli or mezze maniche)
- 300 g of cooked octopus
- 300 g of cherry tomatoes
- 1 garlic clove
- 4 tablespoons of extra virgin olive oil
- 1 glass of white wine
- Fresh parsley, chopped, to taste
- Salt and pepper to taste

Preparation time: 15 minutesCooking time: 20 minutes
Preparation:
1.   **Prepare the octopus**: Cut the cooked octopus into pieces.
2.   **Prepare the sauce**: Heat the oil in a pan with garlic. Add the halved cherry tomatoes and cook for 5 minutes. Add the octopus, deglaze with white wine, and cook for another 10 minutes. Season with salt and pepper.
3.   **Cook the pasta**: Cook the pasta in salted water and drain al dente.
4.   **Assemble the dish**: Toss the pasta with the octopus ragù for 2 minutes.
5.   **Serve**: Garnish with fresh parsley and serve hot.

46.46 Tagliatelle with Porcini Mushrooms

Ingredients (for 4 people):
- 400 g of fresh tagliatelle
- 300 g of fresh porcini mushrooms (or frozen)
- 2 garlic cloves
- 4 tablespoons of extra virgin olive oil
- 30 g of butter

- Fresh parsley, chopped, to taste
- Salt and pepper to taste
- Grated Parmesan cheese (optional)

Preparation time: 10 minutesCooking time: 15 minutes

Preparation:

1. **Clean the mushrooms**: If using fresh mushrooms, clean them with a damp cloth and slice them. If using frozen ones, partially defrost them.
2. **Prepare the sauce**: Heat the oil in a large pan with the garlic. Add the mushrooms and cook for about 10 minutes, stirring often. Season with salt and pepper. At the end of cooking, add the butter and chopped parsley.
3. **Cook the tagliatelle**: Boil the tagliatelle in salted water for 2-3 minutes and drain al dente.
4. **Combine the dish**: Toss the tagliatelle with the mushrooms in the pan and sauté for 1 minute to combine the flavors.
5. **Serve**: Plate and top with grated Parmesan if desired.

47.47 Pasta with Black Truffle and Parmesan

Ingredients (for 4 people):
- 400 g of spaghetti or fresh tagliolini
- 50 g of fresh black truffle
- 80 g of butter
- 50 g of grated Parmesan cheese
- Salt to taste

Preparation time: 5 minutesCooking time: 5 minutes

Preparation:

1. **Prepare the sauce**: Melt the butter over low heat in a pan. Grate half the truffle into the butter and let it infuse for 2 minutes.

2. **Cook the pasta**: Boil the pasta in salted water for the recommended time (2-3 minutes if fresh).

3. **Combine the dish**: Drain the pasta and add it to the pan with the truffle butter. Toss for 1 minute, adding a little cooking water to blend the sauce.

4. **Serve**: Plate and garnish with thin slices of fresh truffle and grated Parmesan.

48.48 **Fusilli with Gorgonzola and Walnuts**

Ingredients (for 4 people):
- 400 g of fusilli
- 150 g of sweet Gorgonzola
- 100 ml of fresh cream
- 50 g of coarsely chopped walnuts
- 2 tablespoons of butter
- Salt and pepper to taste

Preparation time: 5 minutesCooking time: 10 minutes

Preparation:

1. **Prepare the sauce**: Melt the butter in a pan and add the Gorgonzola, cut into pieces. Stir over low heat until creamy. Add the cream and walnuts, mixing to combine. Season lightly with salt and pepper.

2. **Cook the fusilli**: Boil the fusilli in salted water for 10 minutes and drain al dente.

3. **Combine the dish**: Toss the fusilli with the sauce in the pan and sauté for 1 minute.

4. **Serve**: Plate and top with a sprinkle of chopped walnuts.

49. 49 Ravioli Stuffed with Potatoes and Fontina

Ingredients (for 4 people):
*   500 g of ravioli filled with potatoes and Fontina cheese
*   80 g of butter
*   2 fresh sage leaves
*   Grated Parmesan cheese to taste
*   Freshly ground black pepper to taste

Preparation time: 5 minutesCooking time: 5 minutes

Preparation:

1.   **Prepare the sauce**: Melt the butter in a pan with the sage over low heat, letting it infuse for 2-3 minutes.
2.   **Cook the ravioli**: Cook the ravioli in salted boiling water for 3-4 minutes and gently drain.
3.   **Combine the dish**: Toss the ravioli gently in the pan with the butter and sage for 1 minute.
4.   **Serve**: Plate and finish with grated Parmesan and freshly ground black pepper.

50. 50 Spaghetti with Mushrooms and Pancetta

Ingredients (for 4 people):
*   400 g of spaghetti

- 200 g of champignon or porcini mushrooms
- 150 g of diced pancetta
- 2 garlic cloves
- 4 tablespoons of extra virgin olive oil
- Fresh parsley, chopped, to taste
- Salt and pepper to taste

Preparation time: 10 minutesCooking time: 15 minutes

Preparation:

1. **Prepare the sauce**: Heat the oil in a pan with garlic. Add the pancetta and sauté for 5 minutes. Add the mushrooms, sliced, and cook for another 10 minutes. Season with salt and pepper.
2. **Cook the spaghetti**: Boil the spaghetti in salted water for 8-10 minutes and drain al dente.
3. **Combine the dish**: Toss the spaghetti with the sauce in the pan and sauté for 2 minutes.
4. **Serve**: Plate and garnish with fresh parsley.

51.51 Whole-Wheat Penne with Tomato and Basil

Ingredients (for 4 people):
- 400 g of whole-wheat penne
- 500 g of ripe tomatoes (San Marzano or cherry tomatoes)
- 2 garlic cloves
- 4 tablespoons of extra virgin olive oil
- Fresh basil to taste
- Salt and pepper to taste
- Grated Parmesan cheese (optional)

Preparation time: 10 minutesCooking time: 20 minutes

Preparation:

1. **Prepare the tomatoes**: Blanch the tomatoes for 1 minute, peel them, and dice them.

2. **Prepare the sauce**: Heat the oil in a pan with the crushed garlic. Add the tomatoes, season with salt, and cook over medium heat for 15 minutes. Add fresh basil leaves at the end of cooking.

3. **Cook the penne**: Boil the whole-wheat penne in salted water for 10-12 minutes and drain.

4. **Combine the dish**: Mix the pasta with the tomato sauce and sauté for 1 minute.

5. **Serve**: Garnish with fresh basil leaves and, if desired, grated Parmesan cheese.

52. 52 Gluten-Free Fusilli with Zucchini Pesto

Ingredients (for 4 people):
- 400 g of gluten-free fusilli
- 2 medium zucchinis
- 50 g of peeled almonds
- 50 g of grated Parmesan cheese
- 1 garlic clove
- 80 ml of extra virgin olive oil
- Salt to taste
- Black pepper to taste

Preparation time: 10 minutesCooking time: 10 minutes
Preparation:
1. **Prepare the pesto**: Grate the zucchinis and blend them with the almonds, Parmesan, garlic, and olive oil until smooth. Adjust with salt and pepper.
2. **Cook the fusilli**: Boil the gluten-free fusilli in salted water for 8-10 minutes and drain al dente.
3. **Combine the dish**: Toss the fusilli with the zucchini pesto, adding a ladle of cooking water to blend the sauce.

4.   **Serve**: Plate and garnish with chopped almonds and freshly ground black pepper.

53. 53 Whole-Wheat Spaghetti with Tomato and Tuna Sauce

Ingredients (for 4 people):
- 400 g of whole-wheat spaghetti
- 200 g of canned tuna in oil, drained
- 400 g of peeled tomatoes
- 2 garlic cloves
- 4 tablespoons of extra virgin olive oil
- Salt and pepper to taste
- Fresh parsley, chopped, to taste

Preparation time: 10 minutesCooking time: 15 minutes
Preparation:
1.   **Prepare the sauce**: Heat the oil in a pan with the garlic. Add the crushed peeled tomatoes and cook over medium heat for 10 minutes.
2.   **Add the tuna**: Stir in the drained tuna, mix gently, and cook for 5 more minutes. Season with salt and pepper.

3. **Cook the spaghetti**: Boil the spaghetti in salted water for 10 minutes and drain al dente.

4. **Combine the dish**: Toss the spaghetti with the tomato and tuna sauce and sauté for 1 minute.

5. **Serve**: Garnish with chopped fresh parsley and serve hot.

54. 54 Gluten-Free Pasta with Vegetable Ragù

Ingredients (for 4 people):
- 400 g of gluten-free short pasta
- 1 zucchini
- 1 small eggplant
- 1 carrot
- 1 onion
- 200 g of tomato purée
- 1 glass of vegetable broth
- 3 tablespoons of extra virgin olive oil
- Salt and pepper to taste
- Fresh basil to taste

Preparation time: 15 minutesCooking time: 30 minutes

Preparation:

1. **Prepare the vegetables**: Wash and dice the zucchini, eggplant, and carrot. Finely chop the onion.

2. **Prepare the ragù**: Heat the oil in a pan and sauté the onion. Add the diced vegetables and cook for 10 minutes. Stir in the tomato purée and vegetable broth, season with salt, and simmer for another 15 minutes. Add fresh basil at the end.

3. **Cook the pasta**: Boil the gluten-free pasta in salted water according to package instructions and drain al dente.

4. **Combine the dish**: Toss the pasta with the vegetable ragù and mix well.

5. **Serve**: Garnish with fresh basil leaves and serve.

55. 55 Whole-Wheat Linguine with Eggplant and Salted Ricotta

Ingredients (for 4 people):
- 400 g of whole-wheat linguine
- 1 large eggplant
- 3 tablespoons of extra virgin olive oil
- 50 g of grated salted ricotta cheese
- Salt and pepper to taste

- Fresh basil to taste

Preparation time: 10 minutesCooking time: 15 minutes

Preparation:

1. **Prepare the eggplant**: Dice the eggplant, sprinkle with salt, and let it sit for 10 minutes to remove excess moisture. Rinse and pat dry with kitchen paper.
2. **Cook the eggplant**: Heat the oil in a pan and sauté the eggplant cubes until golden. Lightly season with salt.
3. **Cook the linguine**: Boil the linguine in salted water for 8-10 minutes and drain al dente.
4. **Combine the dish**: Toss the linguine with the sautéed eggplant and cook for 1 minute.
5. **Serve**: Plate and top with grated salted ricotta and fresh basil leaves.

56. 56 Spaghetti with Lemon and Shrimp

Ingredients (for 4 people):
- 400 g of spaghetti
- 300 g of peeled shrimp
- 1 untreated lemon (zest and juice)
- 4 tablespoons of extra virgin olive oil

- 1 garlic clove
- Fresh parsley, chopped, to taste
- Salt and pepper to taste

Preparation time: 10 minutesCooking time: 15 minutes

Preparation:

1. **Prepare the sauce**: Heat the oil in a pan with the garlic and add the shrimp. Cook for 3-4 minutes. Add the grated lemon zest and lemon juice, mix well, and turn off the heat.
2. **Cook the spaghetti**: Cook the spaghetti in salted boiling water for 8-10 minutes and drain al dente.
3. **Combine the dish**: Add the spaghetti to the pan with the sauce and sauté for 2 minutes.
4. **Serve**: Garnish with freshly chopped parsley and black pepper.

57.57 Penne with Avocado and Lime Cream

Ingredients (for 4 people):
- 400 g of penne
- 2 ripe avocados
- 1 lime (juice and zest)
- 2 tablespoons of extra virgin olive oil

- 1 garlic clove
- Salt and pepper to taste

Preparation time: 10 minutesCooking time: 10 minutes

Preparation:

1. **Prepare the cream:** Blend the avocado pulp with lime juice, grated lime zest, oil, and garlic. Adjust with salt and pepper.
2. **Cook the penne:** Cook the penne in salted boiling water for 10 minutes and drain al dente.
3. **Combine the dish:** Toss the penne with the avocado cream, mixing well.
4. **Serve:** Garnish with lime zest and freshly ground pepper.

58. 58 Fusilli with Bell Pepper and Almond Sauce

Ingredients (for 4 people):
- 400 g of fusilli
- 2 red bell peppers
- 50 g of peeled almonds
- 2 tablespoons of extra virgin olive oil
- 1 garlic clove
- Salt and pepper to taste

Preparation time: 15 minutesCooking time: 20 minutes

Preparation:

1. **Roast the peppers**: Bake the bell peppers in the oven at 200°C for 15 minutes until the skin is charred. Peel off the skin, cut into pieces, and blend with almonds, garlic, and oil. Adjust with salt and pepper.
2. **Cook the fusilli**: Boil the fusilli in salted water for 10 minutes and drain al dente.
3. **Combine the dish**: Toss the fusilli with the bell pepper sauce, adding a ladle of cooking water to combine.
4. **Serve**: Garnish with chopped almonds and serve hot.

59. 59 Tagliatelle with Pumpkin Sauce and Amaretti

Ingredients (for 4 people):
- 400 g of fresh tagliatelle
- 300 g of pumpkin pulp
- 1 small onion
- 2 tablespoons of extra virgin olive oil
- 30 g of crumbled amaretti cookies
- Salt and pepper to taste

- Grated Parmesan cheese to taste

Preparation time: 10 minutesCooking time: 20 minutes

Preparation:

1. **Prepare the sauce:** Dice the pumpkin. In a pan, sauté the chopped onion with oil, add the pumpkin, and cook for 15 minutes, adding a bit of water if needed. Blend the pumpkin into a creamy consistency.

2. **Cook the tagliatelle:** Boil the tagliatelle in salted water for 2-3 minutes.

3. **Combine the dish:** Toss the tagliatelle with the pumpkin cream and mix well. Sprinkle with crumbled amaretti cookies.

4. **Serve:** Plate and add grated Parmesan cheese.

60. 60 Pasta with Mint and Pea Pesto

Ingredients (for 4 people):
- 400 g of short pasta (e.g., mezze penne)
- 200 g of fresh or frozen peas
- 30 g of fresh mint
- 50 g of grated Parmesan cheese
- 50 g of pine nuts

- 80 ml of extra virgin olive oil
- Salt and pepper to taste

Preparation time: 10 minutesCooking time: 10 minutes

Preparation:

1. **Prepare the pesto**: Blend the boiled peas with mint, Parmesan, pine nuts, and oil. Adjust with salt and pepper.
2. **Cook the pasta**: Boil the pasta in salted water for 8-10 minutes and drain al dente.
3. **Combine the dish**: Toss the pasta with the mint and pea pesto, adding a ladle of cooking water for a creamier texture.
4. **Serve**: Plate and garnish with fresh mint leaves.

61.61 Orecchiette with Turnip Greens (Puglia)

Ingredients (for 4 people):
- 400 g of fresh orecchiette
- 500 g of turnip greens
- 4 anchovy fillets in oil
- 2 garlic cloves
- 4 tablespoons of extra virgin olive oil
- 1 chili pepper (optional)
- Salt to taste

Preparation time: 15 minutesCooking time: 15 minutes
Preparation:
1.   **Prepare the turnip greens**: Clean the turnip greens by removing the tougher leaves and stems. Wash them thoroughly.
2.   **Cook the turnip greens**: Boil them in salted water for about 5 minutes, then drain (keeping the cooking water).
3.   **Prepare the sauce**: Heat the oil in a pan with garlic and anchovies. Let the anchovies melt over low heat, then add the chili pepper and turnip greens. Sauté for 5 minutes.
4.   **Cook the orecchiette**: In the same water used for the greens, cook the orecchiette for 8-10 minutes.
5.   **Combine the dish**: Drain the orecchiette and toss them with the sauce in the pan. Sauté for 1-2 minutes.
6.   **Serve**: Plate and serve hot.

62. 62 Pici with Wild Boar Ragù (Tuscany)

Ingredients (for 4 people):
- 400 g of pici (fresh pasta)

- 300 g of minced or cubed wild boar meat
- 1 carrot
- 1 onion
- 1 celery stalk
- 1 glass of red wine
- 200 g of tomato purée
- 2 tablespoons of extra virgin olive oil
- 1 bay leaf
- Salt and pepper to taste

Preparation time: 20 minutesCooking time: 2 hours

Preparation:

1. **Prepare the soffritto**: Finely chop the carrot, onion, and celery. Heat the oil in a pot and sauté the mixture for 5 minutes.

2. **Add the meat**: Add the wild boar to the soffritto and brown it for 10 minutes.

3. **Deglaze with wine**: Pour in the red wine and let it evaporate. Add the tomato purée, bay leaf, salt, and pepper. Simmer on low heat for about 2 hours, stirring occasionally.

4. **Cook the pici**: Boil the pici in salted water for 6-8 minutes.

5.   **Combine the dish**: Toss the pici with the wild boar ragù and serve hot.

63.63 Trenette with Pesto (Liguria)

Ingredients (for 4 people):
- 400 g of trenette
- 50 g of fresh basil
- 30 g of pine nuts
- 50 g of grated Parmesan cheese
- 30 g of grated pecorino cheese
- 1 garlic clove
- 100 ml of extra virgin olive oil
- Coarse salt to taste

Preparation time: 15 minutesCooking time: 10 minutes

Preparation:

1.   **Prepare the pesto**: In a mortar, crush the garlic with a pinch of coarse salt. Add the basil, pine nuts, and cheeses, continuing to crush. Slowly pour in the olive oil while mixing until creamy. Alternatively, pulse the ingredients in a blender, avoiding overheating them.

2.   **Cook the trenette**: Boil the pasta in salted water for about 10 minutes.

3.   **Combine the dish**: Drain the trenette and toss them with the pesto, adding a bit of cooking water to blend.
4.   **Serve**: Plate and garnish with fresh basil leaves.

64.64 **Spaghetti alla Norma (Sicily)**

Ingredients (for 4 people):
- 400 g of spaghetti
- 1 large eggplant
- 400 g of peeled tomatoes
- 2 garlic cloves
- 4 tablespoons of extra virgin olive oil
- 100 g of grated salted ricotta cheese
- Fresh basil to taste
- Salt and pepper to taste

Preparation time: 15 minutesCooking time: 30 minutes

Preparation:
1.   **Prepare the eggplant**: Dice the eggplant, sprinkle with salt, and let it rest for 10 minutes. Rinse and pat dry with kitchen paper.
2.   **Fry the eggplant**: Heat the oil in a pan and fry the eggplant cubes until golden. Drain on paper towels.

3.   **Prepare the sauce**: In a pan, heat the oil with garlic. Add the crushed peeled tomatoes, season with salt, and cook for 15-20 minutes. Add fresh basil at the end.

4.   **Cook the spaghetti**: Boil the spaghetti in salted water for 8-10 minutes.

5.   **Combine the dish**: Drain the spaghetti, mix it with the sauce, and add the fried eggplant. Sauté for 1 minute.

6.   **Serve**: Top with grated salted ricotta and fresh basil leaves.

65.65 Bigoli in Salsa (Veneto)

Ingredients (for 4 people):
- 400 g of fresh bigoli
- 4 salted anchovy fillets
- 2 white onions
- 4 tablespoons of extra virgin olive oil
- Salt and pepper to taste

Preparation time: 10 minutesCooking time: 20 minutes

Preparation:

1.   **Prepare the anchovies**: Rinse the salted anchovies and pat them dry.

2.   **Prepare the soffritto**: Thinly slice the onions. Heat the oil in a pan and cook the onions over low heat for about 15 minutes until soft and translucent. Add the anchovies and stir until they melt.
3.   **Cook the bigoli**: Boil the bigoli in salted water for 8-10 minutes and drain al dente.
4.   **Combine the dish**: Toss the bigoli with the sauce in the pan and sauté for 1 minute.
5.   **Serve**: Plate and serve hot.

66. 66 Spaghetti with Fresh Tomato and Basil

Ingredients (for 4 people):
*   400 g of spaghetti
*   500 g of ripe tomatoes (San Marzano or cherry tomatoes)
*   4 tablespoons of extra virgin olive oil
*   Fresh basil to taste
*   1 garlic clove
*   Salt and pepper to taste

Preparation time: 15 minutesCooking time: 10 minutes
Preparation:

1. **Prepare the tomatoes**: Dice the tomatoes and place them in a bowl with the oil, whole garlic, basil leaves, salt, and pepper. Let them marinate for at least 10 minutes.
2. **Cook the spaghetti**: Boil the pasta in salted water for 8-10 minutes and drain al dente.
3. **Combine the dish**: Remove the garlic from the tomatoes and toss the spaghetti directly in the bowl, mixing well.
4. **Serve**: Plate and garnish with additional fresh basil leaves.

67.67 Pasta with Seasonal Vegetables and EVO Oil

Ingredients (for 4 people):
- 400 g of short pasta (e.g., mezze maniche)
- 200 g of zucchinis
- 200 g of carrots
- 150 g of fresh or frozen peas
- 4 tablespoons of extra virgin olive oil
- 1 garlic clove
- Salt and pepper to taste

Preparation time: 10 minutesCooking time: 15 minutes
Preparation:
1.   **Prepare the vegetables**: Cut the zucchinis and carrots into thin sticks.
2.   **Cook the vegetables**: Heat the oil in a pan with the garlic. Add the carrots, peas, and zucchinis, cooking for 10 minutes while stirring often. Season with salt and pepper.
3.   **Cook the pasta**: Boil the pasta in salted water and drain al dente.
4.   **Combine the dish**: Toss the pasta with the vegetables in the pan and sauté for 2 minutes.
5.   **Serve**: Plate and finish with a drizzle of raw olive oil.

68.68 Penne with Zucchini, Lemon, and Mint

Ingredients (for 4 people):
- 400 g of penne rigate
- 2 medium zucchinis
- 1 organic lemon (juice and zest)
- 2 tablespoons of extra virgin olive oil
- Fresh mint leaves to taste
- Salt and pepper to taste

Preparation time: 10 minutesCooking time: 10 minutes
Preparation:
1. **Prepare the zucchinis**: Slice the zucchinis into thin rounds. Heat the oil in a pan and sauté the zucchinis for 5 minutes. Season with salt and pepper.
2. **Add the lemon**: Stir in the grated lemon zest and juice, mix well, and turn off the heat.
3. **Cook the penne**: Boil the penne in salted water for 10 minutes.
4. **Combine the dish**: Drain the pasta and toss it in the pan with the zucchinis and lemon. Add fresh mint leaves, torn by hand.
5. **Serve**: Finish with a drizzle of raw olive oil and serve.

69.69 Fusilli with Broccoli Cream and Almonds

Ingredients (for 4 people):
- 400 g of fusilli
- 300 g of broccoli
- 50 g of peeled almonds
- 2 tablespoons of extra virgin olive oil

- 1 garlic clove
- Salt and pepper to taste

Preparation time: 10 minutesCooking time: 15 minutes

Preparation:

1. **Cook the broccoli**: Boil the broccoli in salted water for 5-7 minutes, then drain. Save the cooking water.
2. **Prepare the cream**: Blend the broccoli with oil, garlic, and almonds until smooth. Season with salt and pepper.
3. **Cook the fusilli**: Boil the pasta in the broccoli cooking water and drain al dente.
4. **Combine the dish**: Toss the fusilli with the broccoli cream, adding a ladle of cooking water to blend.
5. **Serve**: Garnish with chopped almonds and serve.

70. 70 Linguine with Cherry Tomato and Oregano Sauce

Ingredients (for 4 people):
- 400 g of linguine
- 300 g of cherry tomatoes
- 2 tablespoons of extra virgin olive oil

- 1 garlic clove
- Dried oregano to taste
- Salt and pepper to taste

Preparation time: 10 minutesCooking time: 10 minutes

Preparation:

1.   **Prepare the sauce**: Heat the oil in a pan with the garlic. Add the halved cherry tomatoes and cook for 5-7 minutes. Season with salt and pepper. Sprinkle with dried oregano at the end of cooking.
2.   **Cook the linguine**: Boil the linguine in salted water for 8-10 minutes.
3.   **Combine the dish**: Drain the linguine and toss them in the pan with the cherry tomato sauce. Sauté for 1 minute.
4.   **Serve**: Plate and finish with a drizzle of raw olive oil and a pinch of oregano.

71. Seafood Lasagna with Lemon Béchamel

Ingredients (for 6 people):

- 500 g fresh egg lasagna sheets
- 300 g shelled shrimp
- 300 g calamari cut into rings
- 200 g shelled mussels
- 500 ml béchamel sauce

- 1 organic lemon (zest and juice)
- 3 tablespoons extra virgin olive oil
- Fresh parsley, chopped, to taste
- Salt and pepper to taste

Preparation time: 30 minutes**Cooking time:** 30 minutes

Preparation:

1. **Prepare the seafood filling:** Heat the olive oil in a pan and sauté the calamari and shrimp for 5 minutes. Add the mussels and cook for another 2 minutes. Season with salt and pepper.
2. **Make the lemon béchamel:** Mix the grated lemon zest and juice into the béchamel, stirring well.
3. **Assemble the lasagna:** In a greased baking dish, spread a layer of lemon béchamel, followed by a layer of lasagna sheets and seafood filling. Repeat the layers, finishing with béchamel and parsley on top.
4. **Bake:** Preheat the oven to 180°C and bake the lasagna for 30 minutes.
5. **Serve:** Let the lasagna rest for 10 minutes before serving.

72. Ravioli Stuffed with Pumpkin and Mostarda

Ingredients (for 4 people):
*   500 g ravioli filled with pumpkin and mostarda
*   80 g butter
*   5 amaretti cookies, crumbled
*   Grated Parmesan cheese to taste
*   Salt and pepper to taste

Preparation time: 10 minutesCooking time: 5 minutes

Preparation:
1. **Prepare the sauce:** Melt the butter in a pan over low heat. Add the crumbled amaretti and a pinch of pepper.
2. **Cook the ravioli:** Boil the ravioli in salted water for 3-4 minutes and drain gently.
3. **Combine the dish:** Toss the ravioli in the butter sauce for 1 minute.
4. **Serve:** Plate and finish with grated Parmesan. Serve immediately.

73. Tagliolini with Lobster and Saffron
Ingredients (for 4 people):
*   400 g fresh tagliolini
*   2 lobsters (approximately 600 g each)
*   200 ml fresh cream

- 1 packet of saffron
- 4 tablespoons extra virgin olive oil
- 1 garlic clove
- Salt and pepper to taste

Preparation time: 20 minutes**Cooking time:** 15 minutes

Preparation:

1. **Prepare the lobster:** Boil the lobsters in salted water for 5 minutes, then extract the meat from the tails and claws.
2. **Make the sauce:** Heat the olive oil and garlic in a pan. Add the lobster meat and sauté for 2 minutes. Stir in the cream and saffron, mixing until a smooth sauce forms.
3. **Cook the tagliolini:** Boil the tagliolini in salted water for 2-3 minutes.
4. **Combine the dish:** Toss the tagliolini in the sauce and sauté for 1 minute.
5. **Serve:** Plate and garnish with a drizzle of olive oil and a pinch of pepper.

74. Fettuccine with White Duck Ragù

Ingredients (for 4 people):

- 400 g fresh fettuccine
- 300 g minced duck meat
- 1 small onion

- 1 carrot
- 1 celery stalk
- 1 glass of white wine
- 4 tablespoons extra virgin olive oil
- Salt and pepper to taste
- Grated Parmesan cheese (optional)

Preparation time: 20 minutes**Cooking time:** 1 hour

Preparation:

1. **Make the soffritto:** Finely chop the onion, carrot, and celery. Heat the oil in a pot and sauté the mixture for 5 minutes.
2. **Add the duck:** Add the minced duck and brown it for 10 minutes.
3. **Deglaze with wine:** Pour in the white wine and let it evaporate. Season with salt and pepper and cook on low heat for about 45 minutes, stirring occasionally.
4. **Cook the fettuccine:** Boil the fettuccine in salted water for 2-3 minutes.
5. **Combine the dish:** Toss the fettuccine with the white ragù and, if desired, top with grated Parmesan.

75. Gnocchi with Castelmagno Cheese and Truffle

Ingredients (for 4 people):
- 500 g potato gnocchi
- 100 g Castelmagno cheese
- 50 g butter
- 1 fresh black truffle
- 100 ml fresh cream
- Salt and pepper to taste

Preparation time: 10 minutesCooking time: 5 minutes

Preparation:

1. **Make the sauce:** Melt the butter in a pan over low heat. Add the cream and the Castelmagno cheese in pieces, stirring until a smooth cream forms.

2. **Cook the gnocchi:** Boil the gnocchi in salted water. When they float to the surface, drain gently.

3. **Combine the dish:** Toss the gnocchi in the cheese sauce for 1 minute.

4. **Serve:** Plate and finish with thin slices of black truffle and freshly ground pepper.